THE RIGI METHOD

by

Sharon Cho

The RIGI Method/Sharon Cho
ISBN: 978-0-9990742-0-6

To Westina, my wife, my partner, my friend.
Without you, this book would never come to be.

Your support is what props me up.

Thank you.

Table of Contents

The RIGI Method: its' Beginnings & Philosophies

Using the RIGI Method

Beyond the RIGI Method

CHAPTER ONE

Welcome to the RIGI Method

Welcome to the "Relax, I Got It" Method, otherwise known as the RIGI Method. To see if the RIGI Method will benefit you, please ask yourself the following questions:

- Do you groan when you get up from a chair or is your back stiff when you wake up?
- Would you like to try yoga but you think your body is too stiff to even consider it?
- Is a pinched nerve or strained tendon, perhaps due to repetitive stress syndrome, restricting your life?

Answering yes to any of the above makes you a good candidate to try the RIGI Method.

Why? Because the RIGI Method teaches YOU to be the driver of self-healing when it comes to tight muscles, strained tendons and other various elements. You are in control of when, where, and for how long so you can say, "Relax! I Got It! RIGI!"

Please note that the RIGI Method is designed to be used in conjunction with other therapies and exercises like yoga, stretching, tai-chi, chiropractic and physical therapies. Using the RIGI Method alone will get you far; however, using it alongside with these other practices will get you much further. For example, sometimes stretching a tight muscle needs weeks before it can fully stretch out. But using the RIGI Method on that muscle will get you there in a few minutes.

Cho

CHAPTER TWO

What is RIGI & How it Can Help You

The RIGI Method is a technique you use on yourself to relieve muscle aches, swollen joints and tendons, as well as other pains throughout your body. But it's more than that. When used properly, it can give short-term relief within 10 minutes. But the best thing about the RIGI Method is when it's used for a long period of time like, more than 3 years. If practiced for this length of time, you can improve your posture, give yourself more flexibility, and even let go of the past.

Combining aspects of Stoicism, acupressure, deep tissue massages, and mindfulness, the RIGI Method teaches you to be more aware of your own body in order to relieve it. You will have the ability to locate tension within your body and using a combination of all aspects, release the stress. Yes, YOU will be in control, hence the name, "Relax, I Got It" the RIGI Method!

The RIGI Method was first developed to relieve pain surrounding a pinched nerve. It was later expanded to include tension knots, locked muscles, muscle aches, pain from incisions and cuts, as well as some rheumatoid and arthritis pain. If you suffer from any of this and are too stiff to try Yoga or stretching, then the RIGI Method is right for you.

If you are someone who can practice advanced Yoga poses, the RIGI Method can still be beneficial. Muscles that have been traumatized in the past can only stretch so far. The RIGI Method is designed to heal old traumas, emotional and physical that are trapped in your body and limits you in some way.

How does the RIGI Method do this? By the following tenets:
- See tension/pain as energy.
- Be gentle but unyielding to your body.
- Let go and relax.
- Breathe in and out, deeply.
- Shake it off.

- Go inside yourself and talk to your body.
- Achieve stillness even with chaos around.
- Remember but don't hold on to the past.
- Apply the RIGI Method into other parts of life

Lastly, please remember, the RIGI Method is a process. Even though initial successes will be achieved quickly, you need to use it for a length of time to get long-lasting results.

Due to the duration of the results, the RIGI Method can end up being a way of life. Once you've loosened and relaxed one muscle, more locked systems will beg you for release.

Think of the RIGI Method as the pathway to a life of flexibility and less tension.

CHAPTER THREE
How RIGI Started

Skip this chapter if your only interest is in how to relieve your aches and pains. However, if you're interested in a direct application of how RIGI works, read on for my story.

First though, you should see who I was before I developed the RIGI Method.

I grew up with severe childhood asthma which put me sick in bed for two-thirds of my life between the ages of 5-11.

Because of the asthma's severity and longevity, for most of my adult life I breathed shallowly, using only the upper regions of my lungs. I had no idea I did this and had always fooled myself that I took deep breaths. Later in life, I slept for over a decade on a waterbed with no support for my back at all, all because I thought it was "cool."

This history translated to locked muscles on my shoulders and around my ribs which restricted movements and furthered my shallow breathing. Contributing more to the mess that was my body, was me being a lousy driver during my twenties and being involved in 4-5 rear-end accidents. The multiple accidents within a 5 year period plus a childhood collar-bone fracture created tremendous trauma in my neck and shoulders. Furthermore, having an uptight personality equated stress in my left shoulder.

8 years ago, something strange happened. Whenever I would cough or sneeze, a lightning bolt of numbness would shoot down my left arm. Concerned, I looked it up on the internet. To my relief, I discovered that I had a pinched nerve in my neck. So I did what most humans did when they find out the pain isn't as severe as they thought.

I ignored it.

Five years later, *after* my wife went through a medical scare, *after* we moved from a condo to a house, *after* we adopted two unruly dogs, and *after* a heavy ladder fell onto my shoulders, my pinched nerve decided it had enough stress.

On the drive to work the Monday after the ladder accident, the pinched nerve flared up so badly the pain bent me over. I had to take three months off work because I couldn't straighten up nor sit for more than half an hour.

In short, my body demanded that I stop everything and take care of it. But how?

The doctors explained that because the opening in my neck was calcifying, the hole pinched the nerve by compressing it. Nothing was going to stop the narrowing over time and at some point, it would close completely. In their opinion, surgery was the only relief. This meant operating near my spine to scrape the opening larger so there'd be less of a compression. A simple procedure they insisted. But because the surgery would be next to my head, I declined.

Instead I searched for alternative answers.

Feeling the area around the pinched nerve proved to be interesting. Everything from muscle to tendon felt clenched and encased in granite. So how could having tight muscles around that nerve be anything but compressing?

Finally I remembered a solution.

When my wife experienced severe abdominal pain due to surgical adhesions, a massage therapist showed me how to break her adhesions up by using deep tissue massage therapy. "Press down with your fingers where it feels firm," she said. "Hold it until you feel the firmness break up." Remembering those words brought up yet another memory: another massage therapist once told me that with a little time, she could cure my rock-hard shoulders.

I had nothing to lose, so I started pressing down on the tightest muscles.

CHAPTER FOUR

Why RIGI Works & What Ailments It Can Help

The main theory behind the RIGI Method is that energy, either in the form of trauma or stress, gets trapped inside your muscles. Because of that trapped energy, you will not find long-term relief until you release that energy.

Here is what I mean.

My muscles got hurt in that ladder accident. (If we ever meet, ask me about this. It's actually a funny story... now.) The weight of the ladder coupled with the force of gravity, landed square on my left shoulder. The impact tightened and compressed my pinched nerve to a point where I literally became disabled.

By using the RIGI Method, I was upright within a week. The muscles loosened up enough for me to move, which in turn relieved the compression. Less than a month later, the pinched nerve screamed less and less.

For those of you who say that time heals most pinched nerves, I agree with you. Nonetheless, using the RIGI Method allowed my healing to be so far-reaching that surgery has been taken off as an option and remains off to this day.

Once I started relaxing those muscles though, I found merely relieving the pinched nerve wasn't enough for me. My body felt awkward because it reached this weird in-between stage of being partially-healed, yet the muscles themselves wanted to return to its old gnarled state where it had felt comfortable for so many years. Think of a tangled phone cord having a hard time returning to its initial neat curls, for those of you who remember phone cords. So, I continued using the RIGI Method to ensure that the healing would stick.

Three years of continuous applications later, not only has the pain from the pinched nerve *not* returned but I'm finally relaxing the knotted-up foundation muscles underneath, next to the shoulder blade. Daily usage of the RIGI Method released enough tension to get in there. The result? My posture is straighter than it's ever been in my whole entire life. The only remnant that shows I have a pinched nerve in my neck is a loss of strength in my left hand and occasional pins and needles running down my left arm.

The reason why the RIGI Method works is because:

- You are in control of your recovery and you can gauge how fast or slow you'd like to go.
- Tangible results come quickly.
- Gentle but unyielding pressure gets muscles to relax, just like deep tissue massages.
- Using your finger for the pressure gives you (instead of a therapist or a tool) the immediate feedback to understand your body better.
- The RIGI Method can be used daily for as long as you'd like, several times a day.
- Learning to let go teaches you to relax more than just muscles.

It's already pretty evident how the RIGI Method can help those who suffer from either pinched nerves or locked/extremely tight muscles.

It can also help with other types of pain, like strained tendons. The idea is similar to how you would relieve muscles but you would need to use a bit more strength. Tendons are less flexible than muscles so it takes a bit more urging. Put a gentle but unyielding pressure on your tendons to the point where they can relax.

Another example would be to use the RIGI Method to help those whose cartilage wore away. Think of a skeleton. There are natural spaces between the joints where cartilage goes. Muscles, nerves and tendons attach to the bones near those joints and nerves pass through empty spaces wherever it can fit. As you get older though, cartilage inevitably gets worn down leaving much less space between the hard bones. Basically, your natural shock absorbers become less effective over time. If you relax the muscles, then there'd be less pressure on those spaces.

The RIGI Method is not a cure-all. What it is, is a method for you to relax any trauma or long-term tightness suffered by your muscles or tendons. But as a result of those muscles and tendons relaxing, you should see positive side-effects like your posture improving, asthma symptoms lessening, and fewer migraines.

CHAPTER FIVE

Where Pain Comes From

The basic theory behind the RIGI Method is that chronic pain in muscles and tendons are caused by residual energy. That energy may be located elsewhere in the body, but the reason you have pain is because of two possible reasons: 1) your body hasn't forgotten the energy of that trauma and/or 2) you are holding onto that energy.

Here's what the RIGI Method means by your body hasn't forgotten the energy of the trauma.

Take for instance, getting hit by a baseball.

In your youth, your muscles will have had very little experience, so the ball's impact will result in a bruise and little else.

When you get older and more experienced, you will react in two ways to pain: ignore it and plow on, or react gingerly.

Let's take a better example, one that I have familiarity with: the common fender-bender.

The first time I was involved in a car accident, my body did not know what was going to happen. As a result, my body was like a rag doll thrown forward against my seat belt. The next few times? I stiffened up naturally! This made trauma in my neck and shoulders much worse but I couldn't help it. I had experience and knew what was coming so I braced for it.

For the next few years, every time I saw a car approaching too closely through the rear-view mirror, I would tense. Sometimes, it was micro-tensing. Nonetheless, those muscles relived the moments from the accidents over and over again until my shoulders became inflexible and tough.

These multiple rear-end accidents also demonstrate holding onto energy.

But energy doesn't have to come from an external source for you to hold onto it. Energy can be generated from you as well and can be formed due to emotional reasons or physical ones.

Emotional reasons are strong stress-filled feelings like anger, anxiety, worry, or fear. These strong emotions leave you tensed-up which tightens muscles. If you are stressed for a long period of time, muscles will get locked into place, which in turn will generate pain down the road. Take for instance, anger.

The Chinese for losing your temper are two characters combined: fire-boil. Why do faces flush when folks are angry? Because the blood rushing there makes your face into a traffic jam and creates energy. Picture a classic cartoon of an angry person: clenched fists, red face, hunched shoulders, and rising steam off the top of the head. Where does that energy go when you calm down? Personally, the energy went from my face and sunk deep in my left shoulder. Which, incidentally, is the shoulder with the pinched nerve.

Let's take another type of emotional energy: self-doubt.

Self-doubt causes all sorts of stress, especially to your muscles. When you have self-doubt, you walk around with tightness in your muscles constantly. Because the muscles aren't allowed to relax, knots build up over time.

Physical stresses are things like repetitive stress syndrome, aging, bad posture, or even sleeping in a bad bed. Sitting all day is another example. To see what I'm talking about, think about any skeleton that you've seen over Halloween. Move the skeleton around like make it have a bad posture, or sit. Now, add muscles to the skeleton. You see how certain parts of the body are stretched, while others are pressed together? Those are physical stresses.

When your body is made to do things like stay in a bad posture or stay stressed for long periods of time, you use energy to make sure your muscles don't budge AND they don't hurt. Over time though, muscles get tired and will weaken. Then other nearby muscles have to adjust and carry the weight.

This is the RIGI Method's concept called tent-poles, where every stress point along your muscles act like a tent pole. Over time, muscles propped up by the tent poles sag and require other muscles to act as tent poles to help carry the weight. Using the RIGI Method will relax your muscles to the point where they no longer act as a tent pole, thus reducing the stress on the other parts of the body.

CHAPTER SIX

Pain Centers As Tent Poles

The RIGI Method's main emphasis is to put a gentle but unyielding pressure on a tight muscle. After a few moments of pressure along with steady breathing, muscles will feel uncomfortable, so uncomfortable that it has to move to not be uncomfortable again.

If you've started to relax some muscles, you should be noticing the muscles' connections to each other. When one part is weak, other parts step in to help be supportive. If you can picture your muscles as tents, then each tension point are tent poles that help with holding up the whole structure but because all the stress and tension are on the poles, they hurt.

So what happens when you take away a tension point?

It's at that moment that you and that muscle realizes it's now possible to relax.

But remember the tent pole theory. Once you've relaxed a muscle, surrounding muscles will hurt, because you've removed that center support and others will have to take up the slack.

What to do then, is to relax the other tent poles.

Here's the good news; while it took many years to get your muscles to where it's all twisted and frozen, undoing the tension takes far less time. Furthermore, after a while of relaxing different tent poles, surprising things will happen.

One example is relaxing some shoulder muscles can make your jaw pop. If you clench your teeth or grind them at night, the pressure you exert isn't confined to your teeth and jaws. It also takes neck and shoulder muscles to keep the jaw clenched. Muscles are connected to each other through the skeletal structure.

To relax the entire body, you will have to work on each of those tension spots in your body, over and over again to retrain your body into relaxing and not curling back into stress positions.

After a while, you will discover one thing: the pain and tightness run much deeper in your muscles than you originally thought. This is when the pain will exhibit its most unusual property.

CHAPTER SEVEN

Pain's Unusual Property

What is the most unusual thing about pain?

Your body gets used to its weight and tries its damnedest to make it seem like you are not in pain.

Most of us can and do get desensitized to the point where we don't even realize we are hurting. That's because pain builds up incrementally AND the surrounding muscles will adjust and twist themselves into a position that changes the pain into a manageable one.

I once touched a friend's shoulder with a gentle but unyielding touch. After a couple of seconds, she pulled away and screamed, "What the hell did you do there?" My first smart-ass thought was, "The Vulcan Nerve Pinch," but I kept my mouth shut. The look of horror at the pain I inflicted with a mere touch silenced me. We were on a dog walk and it was too much to explain that she had locked muscles and that they've been screaming for years; she just hadn't been able to hear it.

With the RIGI Method, you can help yourself to unlock those muscles no matter how long they've been screaming.

Cho

CHAPTER EIGHT

Talk to Your Body

Besides your muscles screaming, your body talks to you in other ways like your stomach rumbling when you're hungry. However, the body sometimes send signals instead like a crick in the neck or a headache that indicates that you slept badly. Your body will even do things like lock up your muscles during a violent sneeze to let you know something's amiss.

In today's society, most of our attention is directed outward rather than inward. Therefore, we rarely understand what our bodies are saying to us. The RIGI Method hopes to train our inner ears to hear what our body is saying when different parts ache, act up or are in pain.

In many cases, aches are telling us we have an old deep bruise from an impact made many years ago. So long ago that we probably forgot how the pain came to be. Or, they're telling you your muscles are tired and worn out from having to hold the same position year after year.

Since your body talks to you in different ways, the RIGI Method suggests that you talk back to your body whenever you are using the RIGI Method.

Don't laugh. It really works. There's something about vocalizing instructions to your body and your body listening.

When you use the RIGI Method, you're listening to your body so intently that in a way, it's similar to meditation. With meditation, your purpose is to empty your mind. If you need to use the RIGI Method, your body probably won't let you empty your mind. So instead, we will focus on listening to your body and trying to understand what it's telling you.

If you groan as you get up, if you wake up stiffly, if you are constantly shifting as you're sitting, your body is telling you it's not comfortable. So sit still and listen to where it's the most uncomfortable. That's where to start.

Once you've begun the RIGI Method, make sure to actually vocalize to the muscle that it's okay to relax. Every time I thank my muscle for a job well done and that it's earned its rest, the muscle relaxes visibly. So give it a try. Tell your muscle there's no need to be on the alert anymore because the danger's passed. Thank that muscle.

CHAPTER NINE

Letting Go

The RIGI Method is so effective at relaxing surface muscles and tendons that users develop a tendency to try it everywhere on a body. The tent pole theory is the main reason why: relaxing the most stressed out part of the muscle isn't enough. You need to work on the rest of the tent poles.

However, there is a phenomenon you should be aware of that happens when you use the RIGI Method on the deeper locked areas of your muscles.

Sometimes, memories spring up.

This is because you released some retained energy from the past when the locked muscle was created. Once, the smell of Johnson's baby powder wafted into my nose. Another time, I heard some pop songs from the 70's. These are the innocuous ones.

Some memories, though, were created during traumatic events. These will pop into your mind when you relax certain stress points in your muscles.

Despite this, try not to be distracted by the memories.

Psychiatrists will tell you to stop and examine them.

Doctors and medical facilities will tell you to get prescription medicines to calm your nerves since these were probably traumatizing events. Again,, that's advice that will keep them in business.

I'm not saying that those professionals don't have their uses. Trust me, I wouldn't be here today if it weren't for those two professions. One gave me medicines to help with my asthma, and the other helped me to better understand my relationships with my family.

But if you are here to learn the RIGI Method, you're trying to learn to let it go. So, do it.

Let the stress go. Allow your muscles and your body to relax.

Yes, there is significance to the fact that releasing your locked muscle brought up visceral memories of the past. But if you give the memories more weight, then you are defeating the purpose of the RIGI Method which is to let things (the past) go. The only significance that you should note is that your muscles are locked, not that that there is a past tied to the stress. Nothing else matters. Let it go.

When your entire goal is to relax, your past's traumatic events will yield to your finger's pressure. I promise.

CHAPTER TEN

Cautions and Precautions

Before we delve into the RIGI Method, here are things to keep in mind as well as some cautions and precautions.

- The RIGI Method is designed to loosen up individual strands of muscles over time. Because the RIGI Method works on the muscle that is suffering the most, what ends up happening are three things that might result in some pain.
  - The muscle learning to move again will cause some pain;
  - The surrounding areas will get strained (See previous chapter about tent poles);
  - Sometimes, memories will get released and often, they're not pleasant memories. This could bring some emotional pain.
- The RIGI Method is NOT meant to be a replacement for Physical Therapy, chiropractor visits, or any medical therapy that you need. It is a supplemental method, designed to help with these other therapies. It can be used as a stand-alone therapy but the results will take much longer.
- The RIGI Method is also designed to be a supplement to stretching exercises and yoga. In fact, the RIGI Method works far better in conjunction with either or both.
- Because your muscles have been locked into position for YEARS, relaxing them means that often you will have no strength in them. Think of someone who specializes in something. Asking them to do something else is inviting an amateur to do the job. This means that when you go to sleep, you might end up sleeping in a different position than usual because your muscles don't know what to do. There is a good chance that you might also wake up with a headache or some soreness in a different part of your body due to the novelty

of your muscles being relaxed.

- Unlocking muscles will cause lots of noises like creaks and snaps in your tendons as they adjust to more flexibility.
- **Do NOT be on pain-killers if you are using the RIGI Method**. Pain is the only way you can figure out if what you're doing to yourself needs a firmer or softer touch. If you're on pain-killers (Advil, Aleve, prescription Rx, etc), do not use the RIGI Method on yourself. It's very possible to over-do things and hurt yourself.
- In summary: there might be days where you are in some sort of discomfort. At that point, you have two choices in front of you: either believe that this is working and continue or be okay with how far you've come along. Either way will bring some sort of comfort.

Remember, it took many, many years to freeze your muscles into position. It won't take as long to get them moving again, but it will take persistence.

CHAPTER ELEVEN

What Now?

You've read this far which means you're interested in trying the RIGI Method and you'd like to get started. So what now?

First of all, you have to get used to one idea.

With the RIGI Method, there is no set way to proceed.

I can sit here and write out a bunch of instructions for different sections (which actually I did do in a previous draft) but I can tell you, you're going to be bored reading them. Why? I was bored writing them.

Basically, no matter what part of the body you're working on, the RIGI Method is the same. You alone decide what part of the area you're going to work on, for how long of a duration and how many times a day. The main reason why there are few instructions is because you will enjoy using the RIGI Method so much that any instructions would almost feel like restrictions.

A few helpful hints:

• Try to balance out the muscles you are working on. If you're working on left muscles, work on the right side after a while.

• Check in with both the muscle you're working on and the surrounding muscles often. You will often clench up during the RIGI Method so check constantly to make sure the other muscles are as relaxed as can be.

• Time will often fly by when you're using the RIGI Method. It's easy to be lost within yourself when making sure this or that muscle is relaxed.

Secondly, you should set up a short-term goal. Perhaps you'd like to get a smashed finger moving again. Maybe you'd like to be able to get up from a chair without groaning. Perhaps you also have a pinched nerve and want to relax the muscles around that nerve to ease the pressure. Whatever your goal is, start small. Once you've achieved that, you can decide if you want to use the RIGI Method for other parts of your body.

Got your goal? Then, let's get started!

The following chapters will give you more in-depth guidance to the RIGI Method.

CHAPTER TWELVE

Here is Where

Okay! Are you ready to start? We will use general terms about the body instead of specifics because the RIGI Method can be used on any aching/painful muscle or tendon.

Here we go.

The first step in the RIGI Method is to identify the area in your body that hurts the most. Even if you know which part of your body to work on, use the following to find the specific point in that area to start.

Sit in a firm chair or the ground if possible. The reason for a firm surface is so your spine and muscles know that they don't have to work hard to help support you. It is possible to use the RIGI Method on a soft surface but realize soft surfaces make some of your muscles work despite the feeling of comfort. Whatever you use as a surface, make sure that nothing is making any of your muscles work. For instance, if you are sitting on a chair with a thin beam across the front for support, is that beam causing your thighs to work? Therefore, make sure the firm surface you're lying or sitting on is the optimum space for your muscles to relax.

Next, close your eyes and breathe in and out, slowly. Go inward with your mind and become aware of your arms, your back, your chest, your stomach, your butt, etc: in essence, all of your muscles.

Imagine what you're touching as rubber bands. At rest, your muscles are supposed to be pliable on touch and without tension. Yet, if you touch some muscles on your body, they're tight. So, are they tight because you use them and frequently? Or are they tight because your body is holding onto some residual tension/energy?

As you keep breathing, examine each part of your body to locate either where pain is or where tension is. Even if you know which area to work on, do the examination; you might be surprised by where the most tension exists.

Often, where tension is, pain also exists. When you first use the RIGI Method, there probably will be several areas that needs attention. You'll need to choose which area you wish to work on first.

To choose which area, you can select:

• The area that hurts the most, or;
• The area that you can best reach. Often removing tension from the places you can get to, makes it possible for you to reach the places you need to get to.

You should do the examination at least once a week because as months go by, areas to work on will shift. Your muscles are relearning how to relax. As they learn, you will need to focus on other areas since they now support the weight that you've relaxed and are probably screaming.

To work on a hand or a finger, press down gently but firmly on the flesh near where the ache or pain is, or where it's stiff. To work on a shoulder, use your opposite hand to press down on muscles and see which one's tight or locked up. Probe along the muscle to find the most tensed up spot. Sometimes, if you press down where it's tightest, an attached part of your body will move, that's how tight muscles can get. If it's your back and you can't reach, please try out one of those plastic or wooden tools that extend your reach like a Back Buddy but remember, as soon as you get to a point where you can use your fingers, do so. The feedback you get on both ends of the pressure is immeasurable.

Basically, find the area you want to work on, probe around gently but insistently to find out which is the most problematic area, then press down gently but unyieldingly on that spot. This is to tell that muscle with a physical presence the place to relax, "Here is where."

Advance RIGI Method

Perhaps, you've relaxed most of the surface muscles and you're having trouble finding deeper muscles to work on. Instead of sitting to find the part of your body to work on, stand.

Stand so that it takes the least amount of muscles to keep your balance.

In theory, your skeletal structure is built so that it is stackable... so that the weight of the head can be supported by the collarbones, the spine, the balance of right to left, by your ribs, by your hips and finally, the legs and feet.

When you stand upright and position your body to have the least amount of muscles working, part of your body will start to ache and perhaps become painful. This, of course, is the place to start. Surprisingly, the sensation could emanate from your stomach around your hip bones.

As always, once you've found the area you want to work on, probe gently but insistently with your fingers to see where is the tightest spot. Then, press down gently but unyieldingly on that spot to tell that muscle where to relax. You are saying with a physical touch, "Here is where."

Cho

CHAPTER THIRTEEN

Be Gentle but Unyielding

Now that you've found the area and muscle you wish to work on, let's get started on using the RIGI Method.

Your finger is far more sensitive than any other person or instrument, so the RIGI Method recommends using your finger (thumb, index or middle) instead of getting something like a Back Buddy. However, due to physical constraints, you may not be able to reach the spot. In that case, use a tool to help.

Usually, a slight pressure will find these spots. Over time, you should be able to find these muscles just by checking inside yourself and without the use of your finger. But for now, your finger is the best way of finding where the stress points are. If you can't get to the problem area, please refer to chapter 14: Beyond Your Reach on page 31.

Basically, the RIGI Method boils down to a few things to do.

- Run your finger along that muscle probing gently to find where it's most tight. Start with that place.
  - You're looking for a part of the muscle that feels firm. There might even be an ache or pain where you press down.
  - Sometimes, what you're working on is so tight that when you press down, the two ends of the muscle moves instead of the muscle flexing where the pressure is.Because of the rigidity, you only have to exert a small amount of pressure to relax that part.
- Use your finger or a tool to exert a gentle but unyielding pressure on the area.
  - How hard to press down is a question only you can answer.
    - Perhaps to the point of discomfort. You use the discomfort to get the muscle to move. I use this

method on my shoulders, arms and legs.

- Perhaps to the point of comfort. Here, you're just relaxing. I use this method to help relax my rib muscles

- Perhaps to the point of pain. Here, you use the pain to let the muscle know it's overworking. I use this method on my pectoral muscles.

- As you keep the finger there, the muscle feels discomfort no matter how hard or light the pressure. Remember, the muscle has had years to be locked in that position and your finger is basically telling the muscle to yield by being an unyielding point. Your muscle will fight you because it's used to being hurt and locked.

  - Remember to keep breathing here.
  - Also remember to have your mind check in with the other muscle around where you're pressing, to make sure they remain as relaxed as possible. If they are relaxed, you can isolate where you are pressing down.

- Spend the next few seconds to few minutes doing three things:

  - Keep up the constant pressure. You don't have to press harder. Just keep it where it is.
  - Remember to breathe despite the discomfort. You will find the muscle wanting to shift and move when you breathe out. So go ahead and move. It's that muscle wanting to relax a little.
  - Actively think about where your finger is pressing down on that muscle. Try to relax the muscle exactly where your finger exerts pressure.
  - Say out loud to your muscle, "relax." (For more information on this, see chapter 16 on How to Talk to Your Body, page 35).

- Depending on how locked they are, your muscles will relax either within seconds or within a few minutes. Either,

  - There will be a very subtle relaxing exactly where the pressure is, which you can feel from both the finger and the muscle or;
  - There will be a sudden, shocking release where more than that muscle will give way under the pressure.

    - Think of this like an avalanche where moving one

stone can unleash a torrent of snow. That pressure on the spot made the whole muscular system uncomfortable and to become comfortable again, all of the connected muscles have to give up their tightness.

- This usually happens to really deeply locked muscles, that have been there for decades.

- When this happens, you might feel an area that feels tight still, that barely moved despite the rest of the muscles caving into relaxation. If so, this is the area to work on next.

• Either continue to work there but move to the next portion of the muscle which feels the tightest or move to another muscle that didn't budge when the whole muscular system relaxed under the pressure from your finger.

• Congratulations! You've relaxed a portion of a muscle using the RIGI Method.

In summary, once you've found a muscle to work on, use a gentle but unyielding pressure on the muscle for a few seconds to a few minutes until you feel something relax. That something could be the muscle itself, or surrounding ones.

Sometimes, you will hear creaking/crunching noises from your muscles. Refer to chapter 20 "Your Body's Reactions" on page 43 and don't worry about it. Just say to yourself, "Relax, I Got It."

Cho

CHAPTER FOURTEEN
Beyond Your Reach

Sometimes because of physical hurdles, it's difficult for you to reach the places on your body that's tight. Perhaps it's because the muscles needed to reach the place are too tight themselves. If so, over time this will rectify itself as you figure out what areas to work on next.

Sometimes the trauma surrounding a locked muscle is too great. If that's the case, refer to Chapter 15 "Having Problems Relaxing" on page 33 where both emotional and physical trauma are addressed.

However, if your inability to practice the RIGI Method is due to your reach (or lack thereof), there are tools that can help.

Please note that the RIGI Method only recommends tools for when it's necessary. The ability of your touch to feel micro-adjustments is invaluable. With a tool, you put a bit of distance between you and your response to the pressure. Therefore with tools, it's possible to overdo things in a manner that may set you back.

So please, be gentle with yourself.

To get to those inaccessible places, you may want to use reach extenders. These tools are often curved with knobs at the end of them to simulate fingers. The curved portion helps pass on more of your strength when you pull down on the tool to assert pressure. The most common of these are called the Body Company's Back Buddy but the LiBa one is fast selling faster because it accommodates more body shapes.

Now that you can reach all parts of your body, what do you do if simple pressure can't get the tight muscles or tendons to relax?

Cho

CHAPTER FIFTEEN
Having Problems Relaxing?

Did you have any problems relaxing any muscles?

If you didn't, continue to the next chapter, "How to Talk to Your Body" on page 35.

If so, read on.

Sometimes no matter how long you keep the pressure up, a muscle just will not relax. No amount of breathing or shifting other muscles can relax it.

In a way, that muscle is "hung up in a memory."

Perhaps a physical trauma caused that muscle to lock up. Perhaps an emotional one. Nonetheless, the important thing here is to get that muscle to relax.

One of the visualizations that helps to "let go" of the past and release these tensions is to imagine the muscles (perhaps think of the rubber band here) being on a hook right where the knot is. You are imagining being hung up.

To be released from this, continue to press down with your finger. Move the surrounding muscles around so that it feels like that particular muscle is being lifted off the hook, right where the finger is pressing down. Did an "ahhh" escape your lips as you felt relief? Use a different visualization if this one doesn't work for you.

If the muscle is still stubbornly clinging to the knot, then you might want to break out the big guns.

TENS (Transcutaneous electrical nerve stimulation) units are often used in physical therapies and chiropractic offices. These devices send small electrical charges to muscles in order to stimulate them, thereby getting them to relax by intermittent contractions. In recent years, portable TENS units have become both affordable and easy to use. Using this machine can reach the deeper muscles to give them the relief they need.

Again, the RIGI Method recommends that you use these when it's necessary. The only reason is because while the electrical stimulation can get the muscle to relax, it's a surface relaxation much like massages. To really get muscles to stay relaxed, you need to use the RIGI Method or some sort of deep tissue massage.

Lastly, if you can reach your muscles and you've tried taking care of the trauma but the RIGI Method still isn't relaxing the muscles, learn "How to Talk to Your Body" on page 35. It really helps.

CHAPTER SIXTEEN
How to Talk to Your Body

Sometimes, despite the ongoing pressure from your finger or a tool and despite moving the muscles around to try and "unhook" it, the muscle will not budge.

At this point, the RIGI Method suggests talking to the muscle or your body.

Talking to your body seems new-age and woo-woo but trust me, it works. Perhaps it's the verbalization of thoughts or perhaps your voice is commanding the muscles, but talking to the muscles and actively visualizing what you want to happen, does help to unlock the tension in the muscle.

What do you say to your muscle when the memory is having difficulty releasing its hold?

First, you tell your muscle that everything is okay and that you're not trying to hurt it when you're putting pressure on it; you just want the muscle to relax.

Next, you *thank* your muscle. It's been doing its job for many years now which was to hold you together, literally. More than that, your muscle was making sure that the skeletal structure and organs nearby do not get hurt. Your muscle's only mistake was not knowing when to stop doing its job. So thank it for a job so well-done that it now gets the vacation it deserves.

Honestly, without your muscles being on the lookout for you, you might have succumbed to some sort of traumatic experience or emotion.

On top of talking to your tensed-up muscle, visualize it relaxing. Instead of a hook, think of a light bowling ball in the middle of a trampoline. That is what your muscle should be doing under the pressure of your finger. It should be that springy and pliable.

Muscles can melt when they are thanked. There can be palpable relief, as if your muscles never knew that it could let go of having to be that stiff of a protection. Try it. Be sincere when you are thanking your muscle for years of service, because it has done a remarkable job. But your muscles are tired and deserves a rest.

For the RIGI Method to work, you need to be tired of holding on to all that stress and tension. You have to want to relax.

CHAPTER SEVENTEEN

Relaxing the Surrounding Muscles

Now that you've relaxed part of your muscle, what next?

If the muscle still feels tight in another part, repeat the previous chapter and continue to work on that particular muscle. Remember to press down with a gentle but unyielding pressure.

But if that muscle's relaxed enough or you experienced the cascade of relaxation, read on.

Previously in chapter 6, "Pain Centers as Tent Poles" on page 11, we talked about how the surrounding muscles are tent poles in their own right. Often, you can find them by searching for probing around the surrounding muscles and finding which ones are sore. Often though, breathing and paying attention to which muscle catches will find it.

Use your finger or a tool if you can't reach them, to press down with a gentle but unyielding pressure on that spot. Keep repeating what you did before in the previous chapter, "Be Gentle But Unyielding" page 27, on the surrounding muscles/structure.

Sometimes, it only takes a few of the surrounding muscles to relax for you to feel so much better.

Sometimes, it takes awhile. Don't worry about it. If you don't have time, continue another day. The work you did today will hold for a few days. But, if you have time, continue to work on the surrounding muscles.

Let go and keep breathing. Make sure your mind is on nothing but checking different parts of your body to see if there is any tightness anywhere. You can use your finger to probe along different muscles. As soon as you find tightness, repeat the method.

When do you stop? Whenever you feel like it. Often, though, the urge to continue relaxing muscles is overwhelming.

Also, be forewarned. It's easy to spend a couple of hours in this mind-space. Those long sessions are tremendously beneficial in terms of unlocking your muscles but you don't have spend that much time each time. Even a few minutes of the RIGI Method can and does help. Five to ten minute sessions can be great, especially when you're driving.

CHAPTER EIGHTEEN
Shake it Off

Congratulations! How does it feel to relax using the RIGI Method?

You are probably feeling a couple of things right now. 1) That muscle and the surrounding areas that you relaxed feel incredibly good. For example, you can bend/move the muscle further than before the RIGI Method and/or 2) all of the other muscles that didn't get the RIGI Method feel constricted and possibly, painful right now.

So, what can you do to ensure that what you've done will stick?

Why, shake things off of course.

Have you ever seen an animal get alert/stressed? They tense up, check out the situation and if there isn't an escalation of tension, they move off to the side and they shake the tension out of their muscles. It's amazing. Rub an old dog and you will rarely feel any knots in their muscles. Why is that? What do animals know that humans have forgotten?

They know that tension and stress should only be a momentary thing. Yes, we humans have the mortgage and taxes and illnesses to worry about, etc. But in reality, does stressing or worrying about those things really ever help? Thinking about it does, but thinking doesn't have tension involved. It's worrying that brings the tension in.

So, literally, shake and loosen your muscles up. It feels great. Shake, rattle and roll!

What happens when you don't shake things off?

You keep muscles in constant tension as you're living your life.

One interesting fact about Bruce Lee, the famous martial artist: the reason he could generate so much power and energy with his punches was because he had complete control over his body. Apparently, his control was so unique he could fire his arm, shoulder and back muscles simultaneously. This was the sudden, shocking power behind his famous one-inch punch.

So, when are your muscles firing?

The horrifying truth is, if you are tense, your muscles don't stop firing. At all.

No wonder I am constantly tired.

So, when you are done with the RIGI Method for the day, take a moment and shake. Shake all your muscles loose and try to keep them from firing unnecessarily. Shake it off.

CHAPTER NINETEEN

Stillness Despite Chaos

A good thing to know about the RIGI Method is that it was designed with today's professionals in mind. That means it's possible to achieve stillness within, despite chaos being around you.

You don't need a designated place to do it. It's recommended that you have a firm support like a hard chair or the ground when you're practicing, but it's not required. Furthermore, the RIGI Method can be practiced almost anywhere: in your car, on the subway, at your desk, out in the woods, anywhere!

You don't need silence to practice it. You should be able to practice the RIGI Method on the couch while the dogs are barking at the mail-woman. All that's needed is the ability to go inward and focus on what your muscles are doing.

Specific clothing isn't needed either. If you're comfortable in loose clothing, by all means. If tighter clothing is better, great! The only thing that's asked is that the clothing isn't restrictive like girdles or really tight bikini string tank tops. The idea is to get your muscles to relax, not tighten.

Any time you feel that part of your body is stiff, check that particular muscle out. For instance, do you hold your breath when you exert yourself? If so, feel around your body to see which is the tightest when you hold your breath. Sometimes a slight pressure is enough to let the muscle know that it's tightened up and it needs to relax. And it only takes a moment.

The only thing to be aware of is that sometimes when you're unlocking your muscles, you have to move your limbs or torso around relieve the tightness. This means that you might swing your arm around just to get a shoulder muscle to relax. When that happens in a crowded subway or a fancy restaurant, you could get some stares. Trust me. I've experienced it.

We encourage people to try the RIGI Method no matter where they are, whether you're at home, the office, the middle of bumper-to-bumper traffic, or in the middle of a field. Go use it so you can say, "Relax! I Got It!"

CHAPTER TWENTY
Your Body's Reactions

During sessions using the RIGI Method, a few things might happen: 1) your body can generate a ton of heat when it is about to relax something that has been held tight for many years, 2) your body can make noises and 3) sometimes, relaxing a muscle or tendon that's been locked into place for decades can hurt.

Whenever your body is about to release long-held tension, it will heat up and you will sweat. This is part of the healing process. Think of your body as tearing itself away from its long-term duty. Those muscles have held your skeleton in place for years. You are telling that muscle to unclench.

Have you ever held anything for a long time? Hours? When you release that object, doesn't it take a moment for your muscles to ease back into a relaxed state? Therefore, it's that much harder when they've been doing the same job for years. So welcome that feeling of sudden heat. It means you're about to get back some energy.

The other thing your body will do during sessions of the RIGI Method is make creaking and popping noises, just like at the chiropractor's. The difference is, the chiropractor is manipulating and forcing realignments which causes the pops. With the RIGI Method, the noises come from your muscles and tendons learning to lose tension.

Aside from noises and sweat, sometimes it's painful to relax a muscle especially when you get to the deeper muscles. Just keep breathing and rub that area after it's relaxed a little.

Sometimes as I described in an earlier chapter, using the RIGI Method will cause your muscles to relax suddenly in a cascading manner, like an avalanche of relaxation. Sharp pain can accompany the avalanche as your muscle panics. The pain should fade within seconds and go away within a minute or two. Just remember to keep breathing to get all the muscles to

Cho

relax.

This cascading effect often will lead you to the next part of the body that you want to work on because part of your muscle structure probably did not relax. Think of snow ridges created by avalanches; somehow miraculously, they are still precariously perched. Your still-tight muscles are like these ridges and need your help to loosen them up.

These reactions from your body are ways to tell you that yes, the RIGI Method is working. So, keep saying to yourself, "Relax! I Got It!"

CHAPTER TWENTY-ONE
How to Know When to Stop

After a while of using the RIGI Method, how do you know when to stop?

Well, have you achieved your initial goal? Then maybe it's time.

Basically, it's up to you when to stop. Maybe you need a break from being mindful of your body to this degree. Perhaps, five minutes is all you can do which can still undo months to years of tightness; it just takes a longer time.

However, be forewarned: the RIGI Method is addicting.

You could end up practicing a little RIGI whenever you sit or stand, simply because you're now aware of what your muscles are doing or not doing. Or, you could end up staring at someone but not see them because you're lost inside yourself trying to relax that *one* muscle, not that that's happened to me. Nope.

In short, you can use the RIGI Method for as long as you'd like, even if it's only for a few minutes.

As for when to stop using the RIGI Method? That really depends on if you had goals when you started. Are you able to move more freely now? Has what sent you here in the first place been taken care of? Have you gotten the flexibility you wanted?

If so, maybe it's time to stop.

But if the RIGI Method has shown you that there are deeper layers yet to be unlocked, you may wish to continue beyond your initial goals and more. The RIGI Method could end up becoming a way of life.

Cho

CHAPTER TWENTY-TWO

The Present isn't Important

Because the RIGI Method uses Stoicism as one of its foundations, usage can extend beyond your physical body.

One thing being constantly reiterated throughout this book is energy trapped inside your body is a reason why your muscles are tight or locked up. Sometimes when you use the RIGI Method, muscles relaxing will release energy. Most of the time, it's physical and appears as heat which makes you sweat. But sometimes, the released energy appears as memories.

How does this happen? As traumatic events happen, your heightened emotions like anger or fear or anxiety get trapped inside the tight muscles. So if you didn't shake the energy off afterwards, the energy stays within and petrifies into pain a few years later. When you release these muscles, you might smell something from the past, or feel some deep emotions.

In time, you learn that in order to prevent these current traumatic events from becoming problems in the future, you need to learn to let them go now. You learn to stay in a relaxed state because otherwise, all the great work you've been doing with the RIGI Method gets undone.

You learn to only take on the important things and even then, not let that energy reside within.

Besides, your body will enjoy being relaxed more than tense, so you will feel in subtle ways that you're tightening up. If you don't hear it, your body will get louder, trust me.

This is why as you use the RIGI Method more and more in life, that you'll opt not to get tensed up in the first place. The present isn't so important that you need to remember it in your muscles years later.

CHAPTER TWENTY-THREE

Getting to Where Life has to Change

Using the RIGI Method and letting go of the past will get you far with regards to relaxing muscles. At some point however, your progress might hit a wall.

There might be several reasons for this.

- It could be because an external object in your life is holding back your progress.
- Perhaps you don't have the strength in the parts that you've relaxed, to help support the rest of your body.
- Possibly you can't, for all sorts of legitimate reasons, get past the trauma that's left in your body.
- Or there's no more to be done. You've done the absolute most already because of the physical damage done to your body.

The important thing is to recognize if any of the above is your obstacle, or whether you're just spinning your wheels with the RIGI Method and need to get other help.

Sometimes, an external object could be holding you back.

Here's an example. A pinched nerve in the neck put me on disability for 3 months. For two years, I used the RIGI Method and got myself to the point my pinched nerve no longer was an everyday concern and I felt looser.

After a while though, I used the RIGI Method to claw back what was undone during the middle of the night instead of gaining progress on my healing. At first I thought it was the technique. Then after a careful evaluation of my life and lifestyle, I realized it was how I slept.

At that time, I was sleeping on a very soft, memory-foam bed which provided little to no support for either my neck or my back. Switching to a buckwheat pillow gave much more support to my neck and helped. But, progress again slowed to a halt a few months later.

About that time, I read about the Ultimate Earth Bed which is a literal sand bed: a mattress filled with sand. I realized this bed perfectly epitomized the RIGI Method's precept: gentle but unyielding. So I went out the next weekend and got it despite having to travel 400 miles to get it.

What this bed has done is give my spine and skeletal structure enough support that my muscles do not have to work much when I'm sleeping. Now, because I can sleep through the night, my progress continues and I barely have any pain when I wake up. Also because the bed is so firm, I can use it to do the RIGI Method on my lower back.

Please note that this was my solution but it may not be yours. You have to be the one to examine your life and lifestyle to figure out what changes could and should be made. Or, make an appointment with me (either in person or through video chat) and I can make a home-inspection. This inspection ensures that your seating and sleeping arrangements at home give your muscles a chance to be the most relaxed.

Another reason for the stall in progress could be that your current strength in the parts that you've relaxed might not be enough to support the rest of your body. Having non-existent strength in my back and neck, I had to do strengthening exercises to prevent setbacks after I got the muscles to relax. If your muscle has been doing the same thing for the past 20-30 years, it's weak when you ask it to do anything else.

Still another reason your progress could be halted may be because the trauma that started the pain is just too great for you to overcome with the RIGI Method. In this case, please consult with a medical doctor or some other expert to get further in your treatment.

Sometimes, our muscles are locked because of PTSD. Some past trauma so affected you that your muscles remain in constant stress. And you want relief from that stress.

Be aware that you may or may not be in the right mind-space to get rid of the traumatic past. If you are, please work with a professional to get past the traumatic events. If you aren't ready yet, I'm sorry but there's a limit to what the RIGI Method can do. Just know that the RIGI Method is here for you to pick up again, once you're ready to let go.

Lastly, your progress may be halted because of physical limitations.

For example: I can never regain the strength in my left hand that's been affected by the pinched nerve. The most I can do is ensure that there is less stress on the nerve, so that there is less pain. I can also try to reduce the loss of strength in those affected fingers.

Because of all these reasons listed above, your progress could be halted. But you can always start up the RIGI Method when you make adjustments, whether that's changing your physical surroundings or seeking professional help like a psychiatrist or a medical doctor.

With these changes, you could be saying once again, "Relax! I Got It!"

If you liked what you read, please go to RIGIMethod.com for links to review the book. Thanks!

CHAPTER TWENTY-FOUR
Helpful Products

The RIGI Method can use some help along the way. Sometimes, rubbing an oil that heats up your muscle is just what that muscle needs. Or perhaps your bed no longer supports how your body is reshaping.

These are products that might be helpful.

- Ultimate Earth Bed - This bed is made from sand, animal skins and latex. It's the first of its kind, a sand-bed. The sand provides the firmness while the animal skins provide the gentleness which is in keeping with the RIGI Method's motto: gentle but unyielding.
- Bucky, the Buckwheat pillow - These are great support for your neck when you sleep or when you travel. Again, these types of pillows are the epitome of "gentle but unyielding."
- White Flower Oil - Great for sore muscles! Rub it on and then let the heat relax you.

You can find more products on RigiMethod.com under "Thoughts & Reviews."

CHAPTER TWENTY-FIVE
Sharon Cho's Background

In my youth, I had such bad childhood asthma that I was sent to an old kung-fu master in Singapore. He was one of the most amazing men I had ever worked with. Despite his advanced age (He was in his 70's), his strength surpassed that of his disciples. He taught me that most things in the human body was pliable: to clear my throat of phlegm, he'd push his fingers from one front side of my esophagus back until he could feel my spine, then he'd let go and all the phlegm would magically disappear... for a while.

We explored different healing energies, from using pressure on different points on the head to checking the muscles' flexibilities in the hands. His efforts relieved me of so many different ailments from migraines to asthma, but before I could fully pledge to be his disciple, I emigrated to the US.

Another influence was a deep tissue massage therapist who taught me how to break up my wife's surgical adhesions because we were too poor to pay for the massages. She taught me how to hold firm until the adhesions tore to give her more flexibility and less pain.

My last influence was studying Stoicism. For stoics, you have to stay in the present and act as if there is no tomorrow.

Finally, I paid attention to what my body was doing, what my reactions were and how I could get past my own self towards self-healing. This is how the RIGI Method developed over a three-year period.

My physical therapists were astounded with the level of self-healing I achieved. "It's very hard to heal yourself," they said. Of course, I don't believe them, which is why I'm bringing the RIGI Method to you. So you can help yourself to say, "Relax! I Got It!."

The End

www.ingramcontent.com/pod-product-compliance
Lightning Source LLC
Chambersburg PA
CBHW071933020426
42331CB00010B/2854